Reiki Rickie shares ReikiKids ™

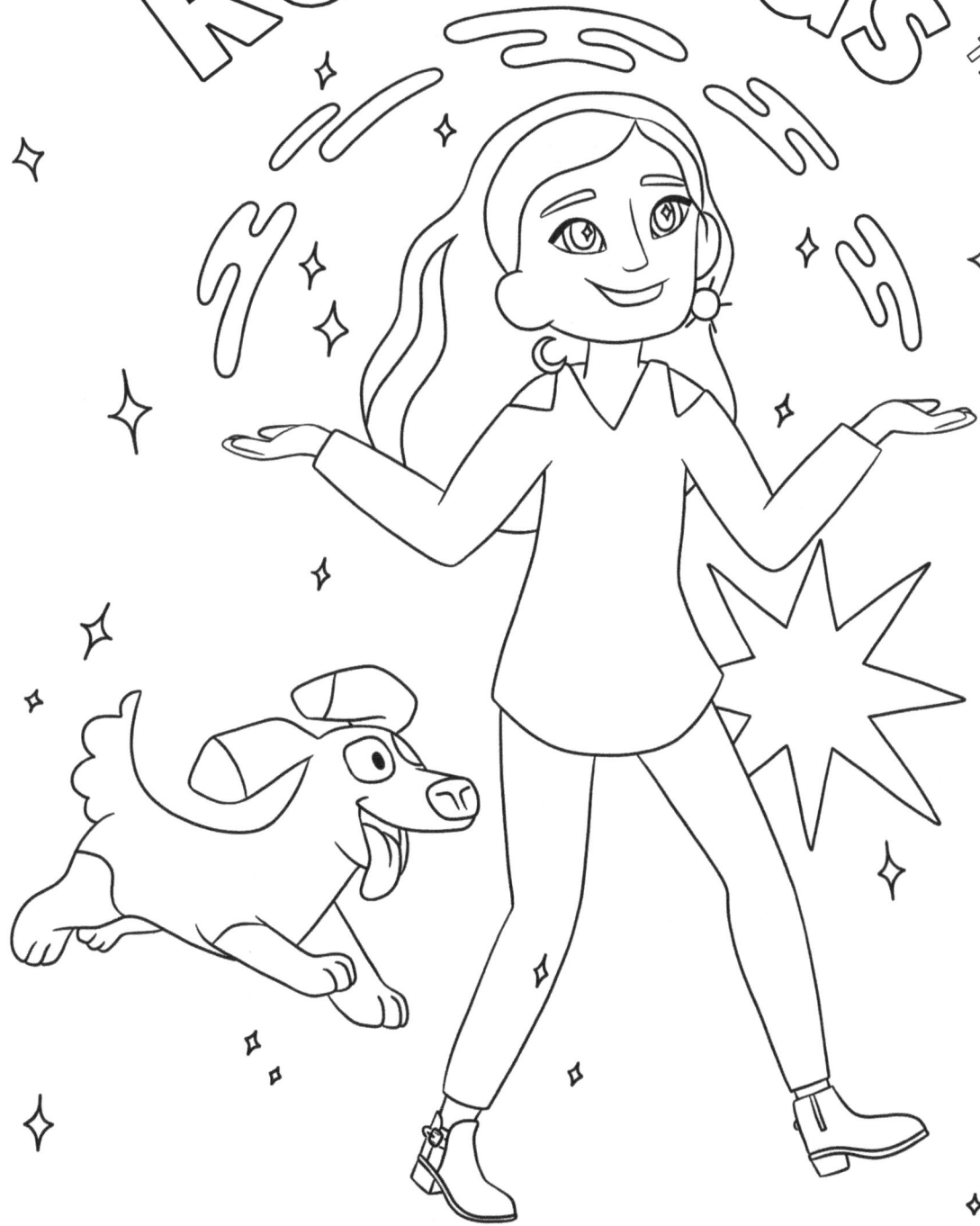

INTRODUCING REIKI RICKIE AND FLUFFY PUPPY

This book is Inspired by and created for the memory of my son Ryan Matthew Daniels. The original "Fluffy Puppy", who still helps me teach Reiki, was his stuffed animal.

This book is Dedicated to more Peace, Kindness, Compassion and Understanding in the world starting with ReikiKids everywhere!

ISBN: 978-0-578-68962-3

www.ReikiByRickie.com

Written by Rickie Freedman and Illustrations by Sarah Massie
Printed in China.

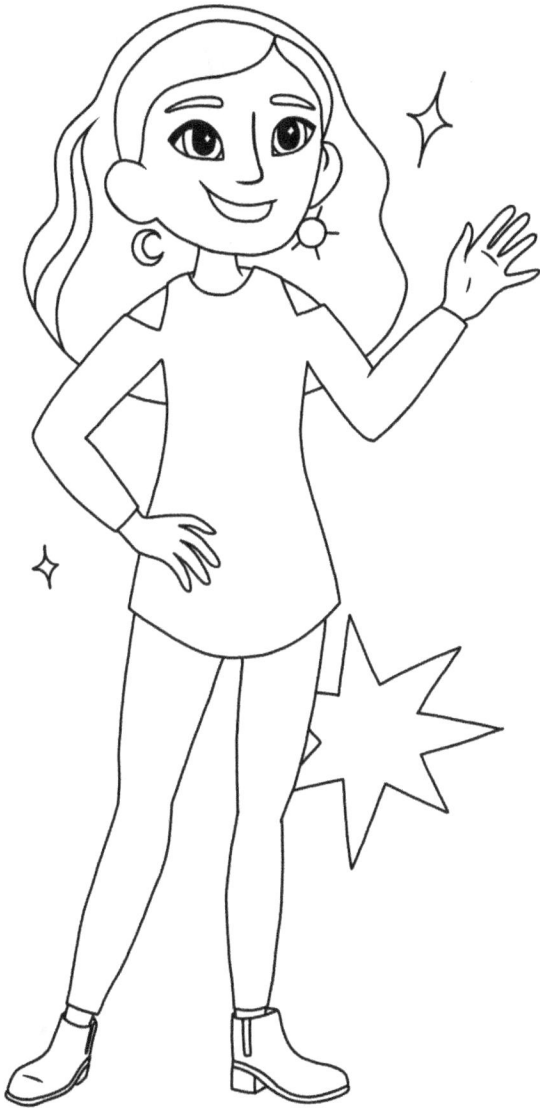

"HI! I am so excited to share Reiki with you, and help you learn all about your energy!

Reiki is for EVERYONE!"

**DRAW YOUR NAME BELOW
AND COLOR IT IN WITH YOUR FAVORITE COLOR!**

Getting to know YOU

TELL ME SOMETHING YOU LIKE MOST ABOUT YOURSELF

I am _____

_____

_____

I feel HAPPY when _____

_____

_____

I feel at PEACE when _____

_____

_____

I want to HELP when _____

_____

_____

One of my GIFTS is _____

_____

_____

Meet my favorite animal

Fluffy!

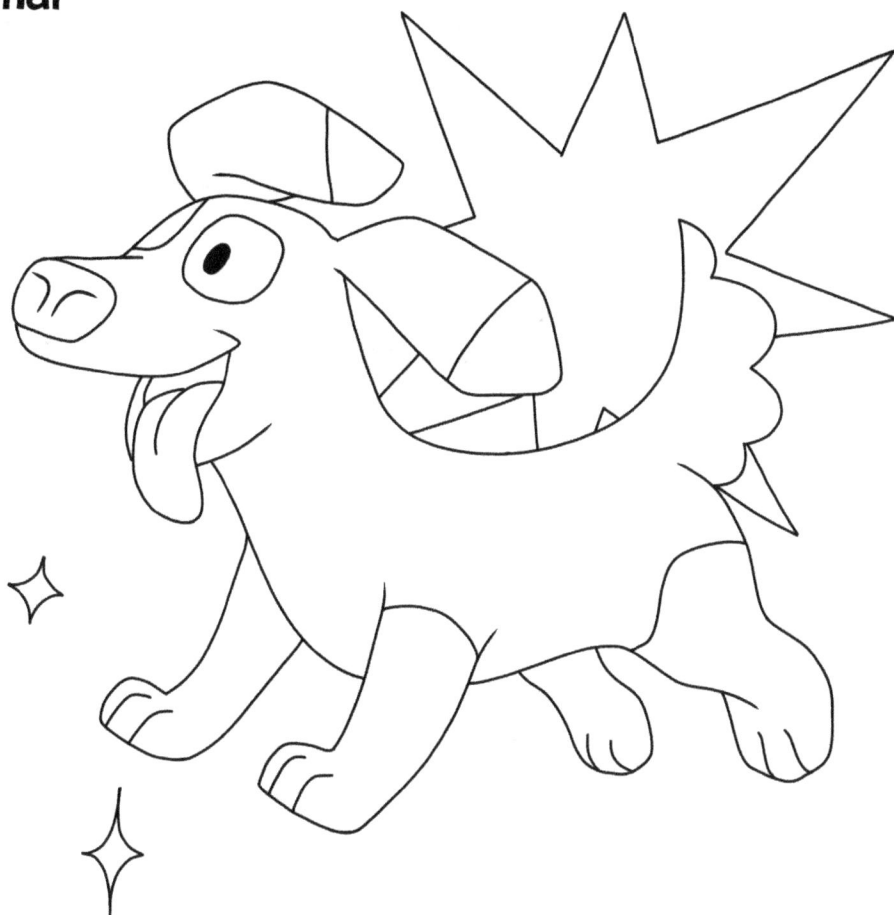

DRAW YOUR FAVORITE ANIMAL

What is Reiki?

(Pronounced RAY-KEY)

DRAW A BIG SUNSHINE   **DRAW A BIG KEY**

➕

Reiki is like the warmth and light of the sun and
is the KEY to all the Love in your heart.

With practice, you can use this energy for healing.
You can spread goodness and kindness to help make the world a better,
safer, more peaceful, and more loving place.

DRAW A PICTURE OF THE GLOBE SURROUNDED BY PEACE AND LOVE

Reiki was from Japan and is now shared all over the world. It is a Healing Energy that comes through us and can be shared through the palms of your hands for yourself, and to help your family and pets.

TRACE YOUR LEFT HAND AND IN THE MIDDLE DRAW LIGHT COMING OUT OF THE CENTER

TRACE YOUR RIGHT HAND AND IN THE MIDDLE DRAW
LOVE COMING OUT OF THE CENTER

ENERGY
Everything is made of energy... including us!

HIGH ENERGY

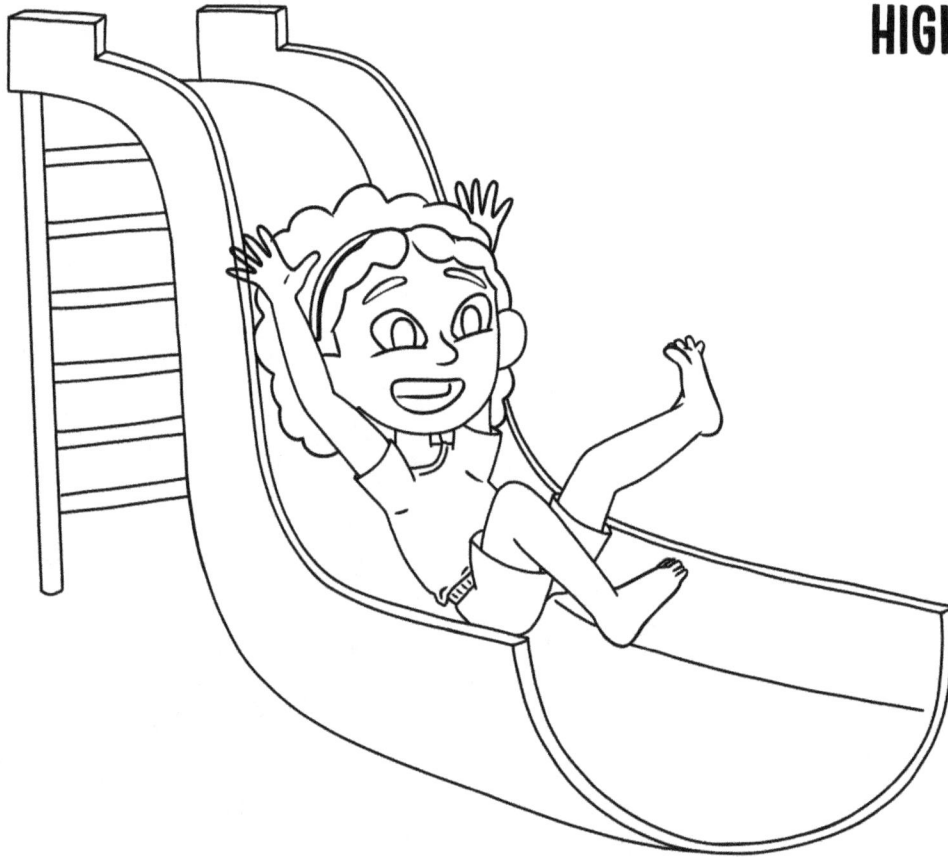

What are some PHYSICAL examples of high energy?
Reiki Rickie Loves to DANCE! _____

_____

_____

What are some EMOTIONAL examples of high energy?
Reiki Rickie Chooses LOVE. _____

_____

_____

LOW ENERGY

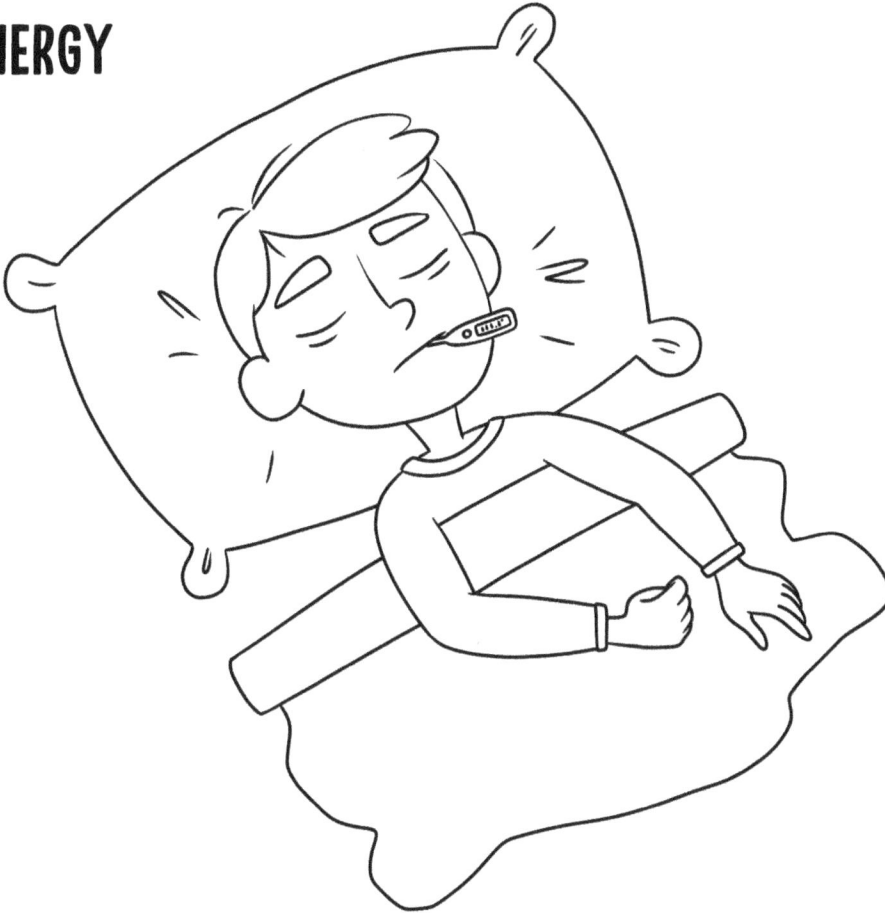

What are some PHYSICAL examples of low energy?
Fluffy Puppy feels low energy when he is too tired.

_____

_____

What are some EMOTIONAL examples of low energy?
Fluffy Puppy feels low energy when he is angry or sad.

_____

_____

LET'S FEEL OUR ENERGY!

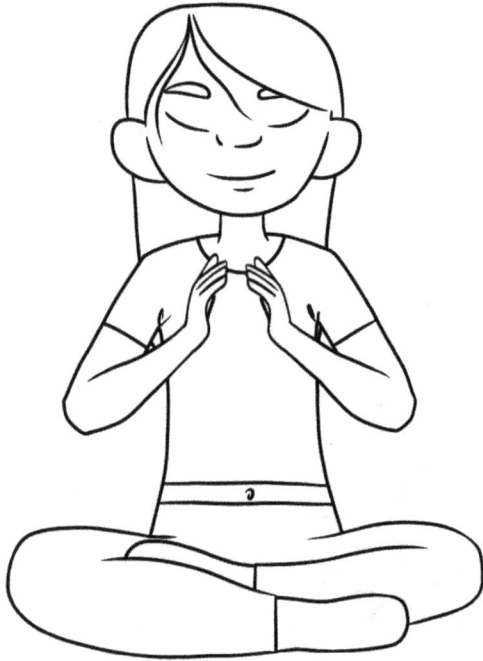

Feel the energy from you

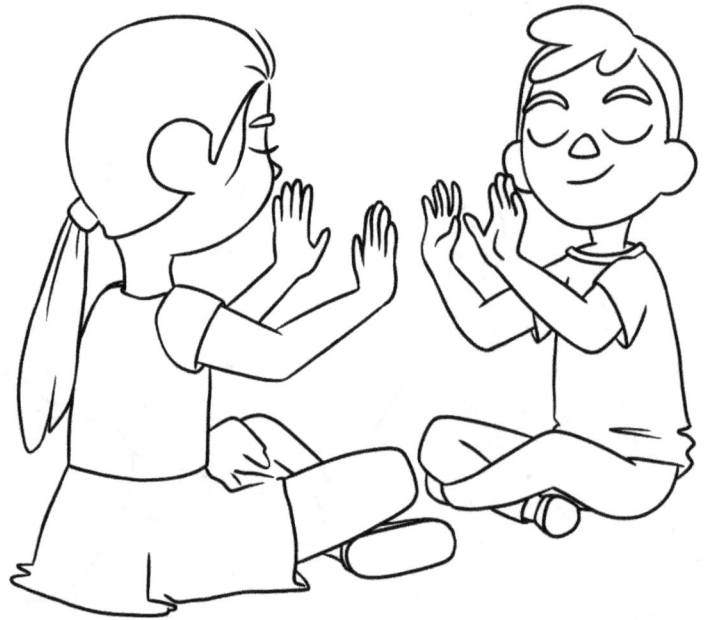

Feel each other's energy

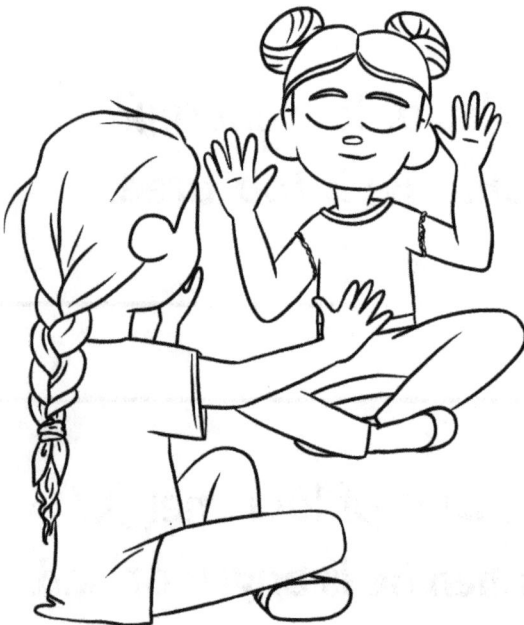

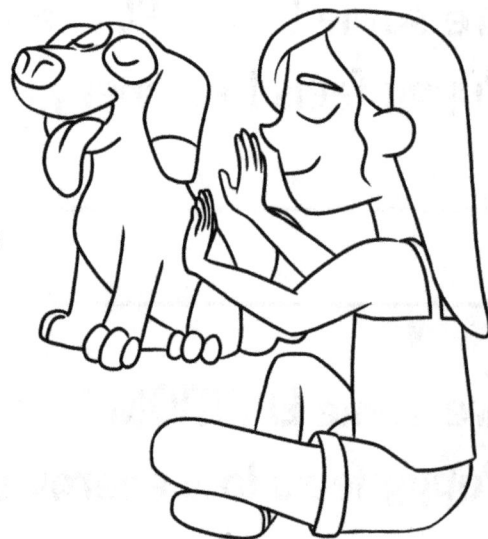

When we work together, we can put more loving
energy into the world!

Reiki History

Reiki was discovered by Mikao Usui from Japan. He wanted to study and learn how people could help heal each other. After reading lots of books and talking with many teachers, he still didn't feel that he knew the whole answer.

He decided to climb a mountain and meditate to learn about the energy.

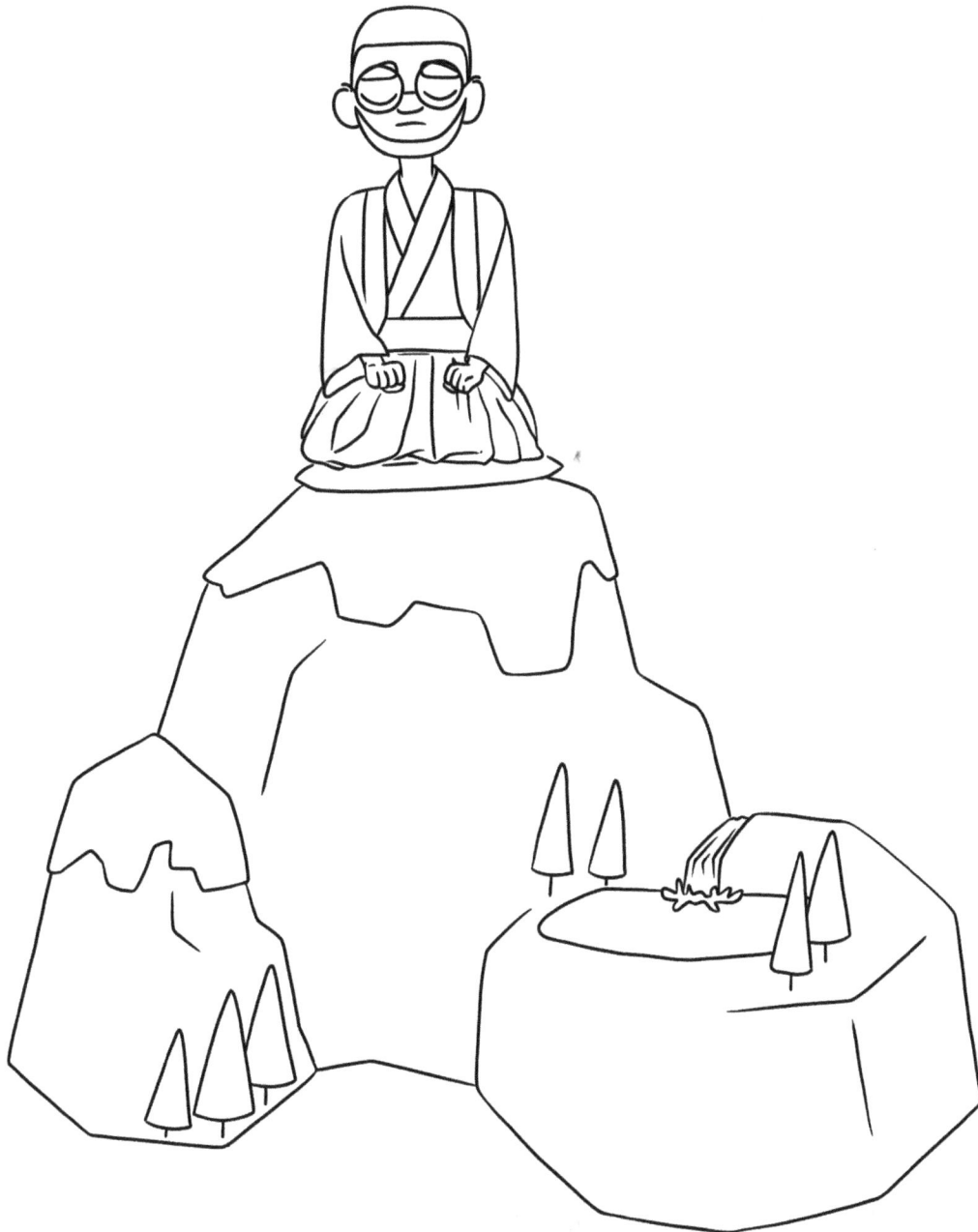

Sitting, breathing, and being still is called MEDITATING.

LET'S PRACTICE MEDITATING!
CAN YOU SIT STILL WITH YOUR EYES CLOSED BREATHING IN AND OUT FOR ONE MINUTE?

Mikao Usui meditated on top of the mountain for 21 days. That's a long time!

Each day he added a rock to a pile to help him keep track of the time.

DRAW 21 ROCKS ON A PILE BELOW

Mikao Usui didn't eat for 21 days. That took a lot of patience! On the 21st day he received the gift of Reiki and came down the mountain.

WHAT USUI LEARNED ABOUT REIKI

Mikao Usui learned about his energy including how to help himself heal, and how to share Reiki with others. He also developed the Reiki Principles to help remind us that we can LIVE Reiki too!

Reiki Healing Principles

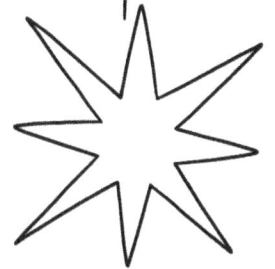

JUST FOR TODAY...I WON'T WORRY

JUST FOR TODAY...I WON'T GET ANGRY

I WILL BE KIND TO EVERYONE

I WILL DO MY WORK HONESTLY

I AM GRATEFUL FOR ALL MY BLESSINGS

RECEIVING THE GIFT OF REIKI

The ability to use Reiki is transferred to your hands through a Reiki Master in a special ceremony called an Attunement.
It helps you remember that you are connected to the source of Reiki, allows it to flow through you, and allows you to use it for healing yourself and others.
We are all made of Energy!

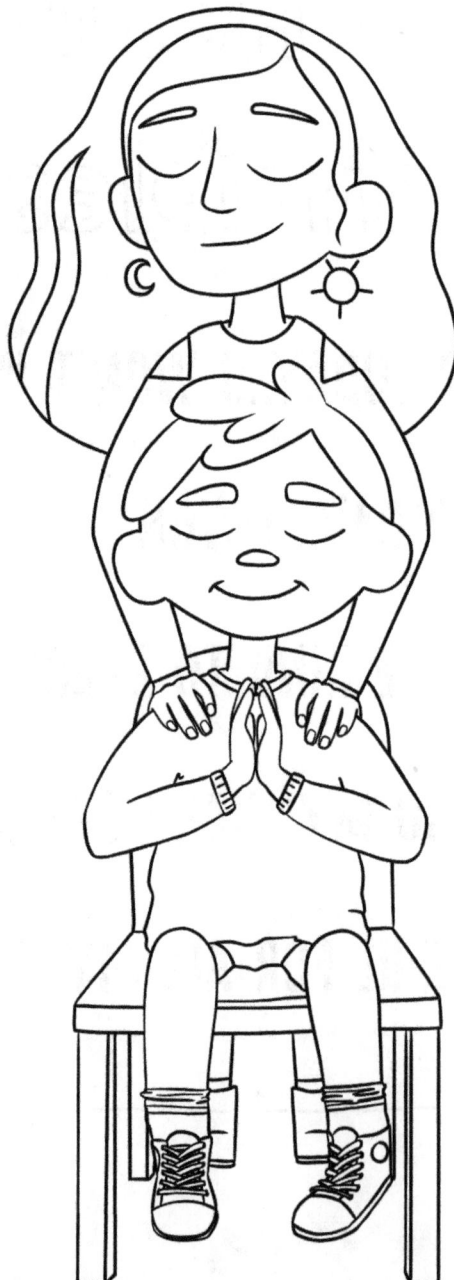

You can do Reiki on yourself

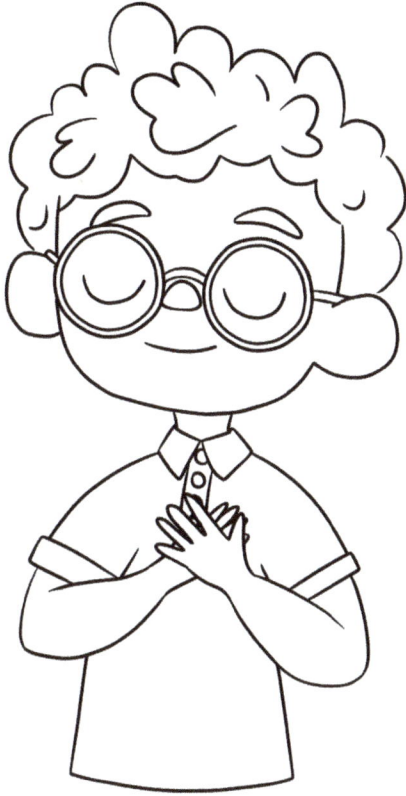

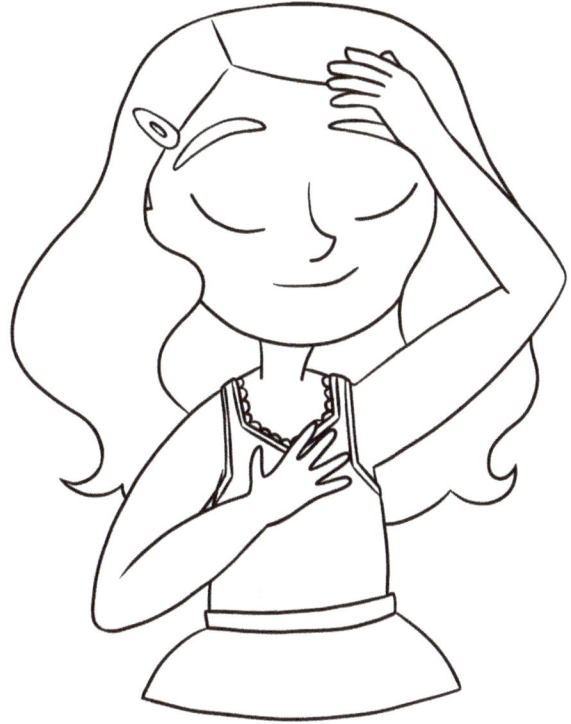

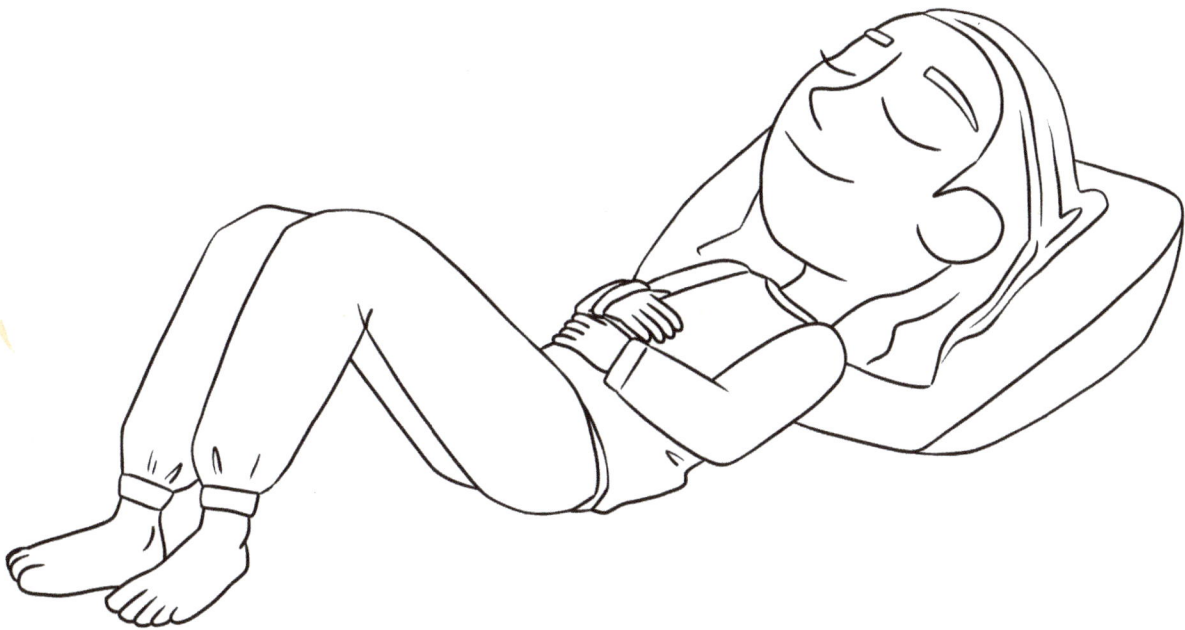

Always fill yourself up first!

You can share Reiki with your friends and family

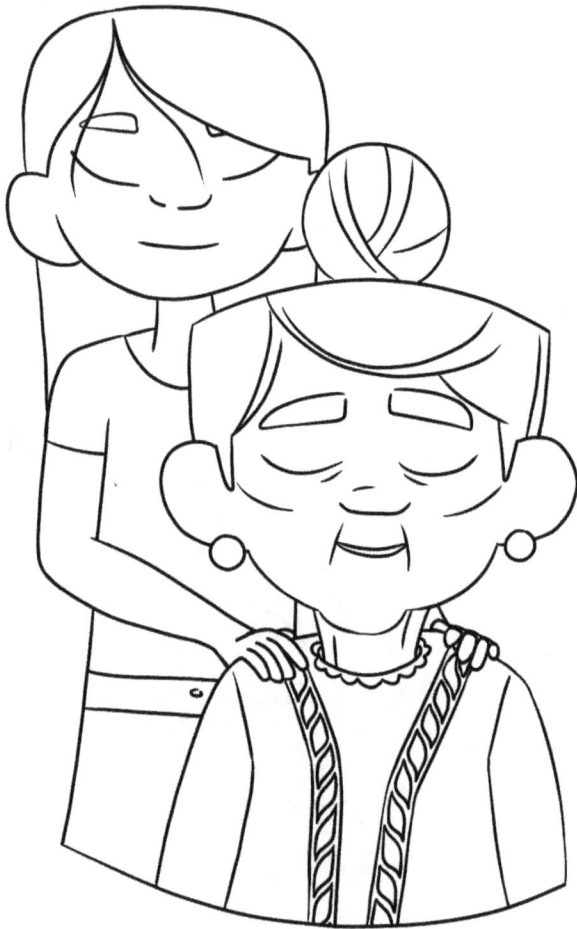

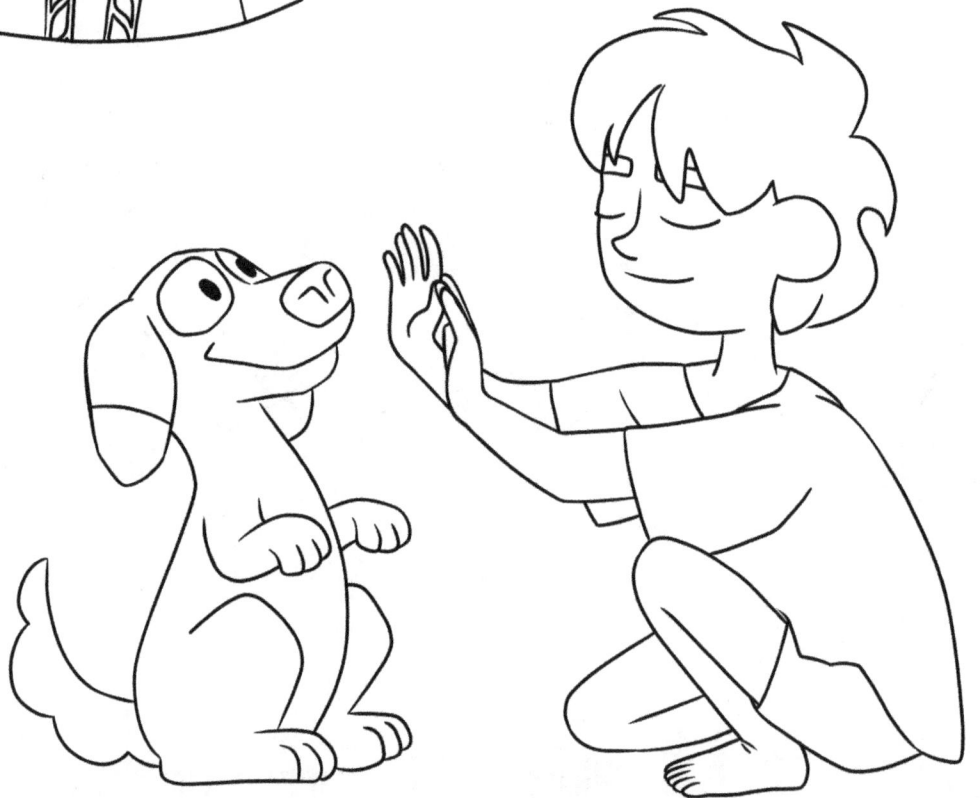

You can use Reiki on plants

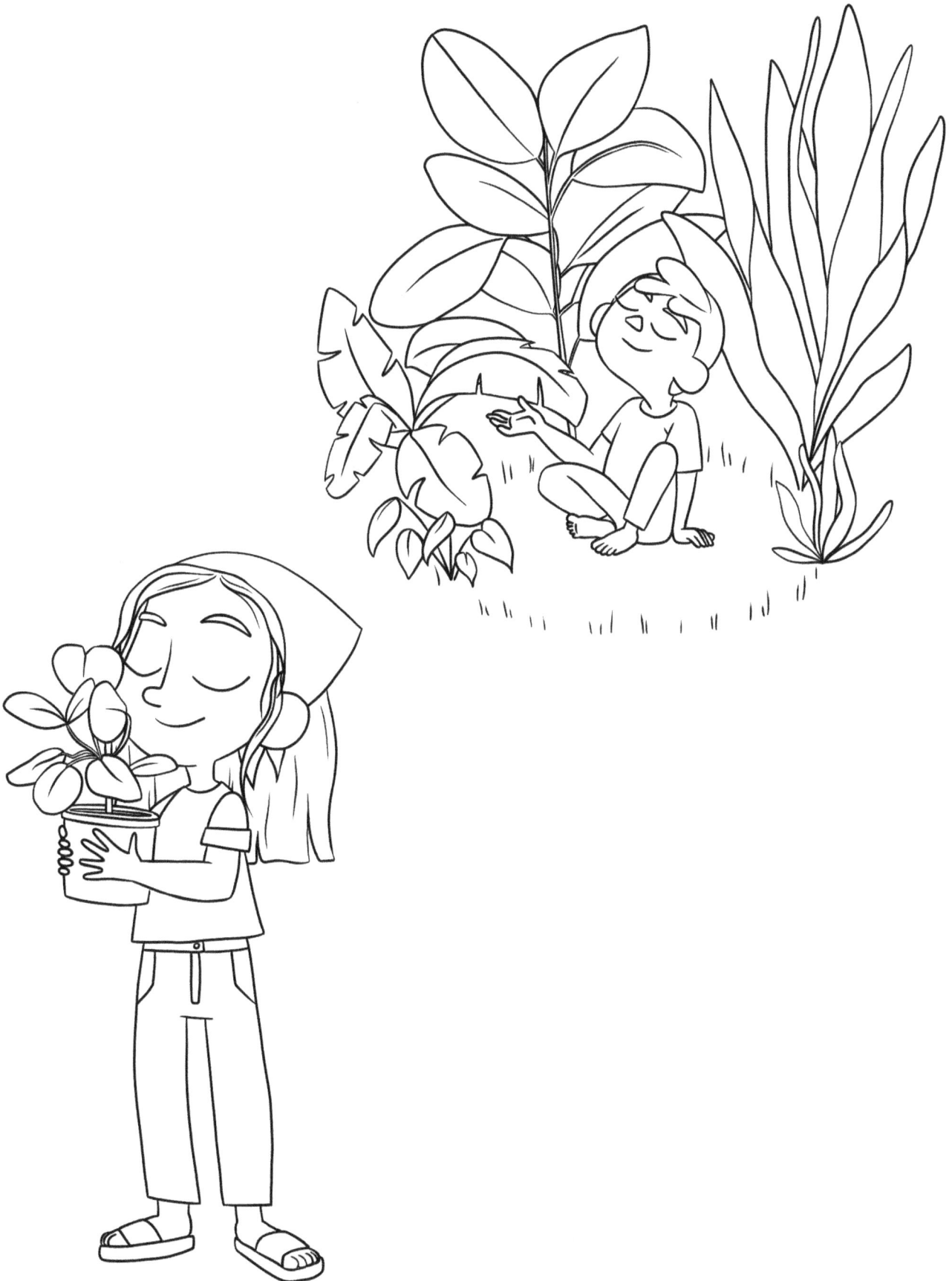

You can share Reiki with your pets

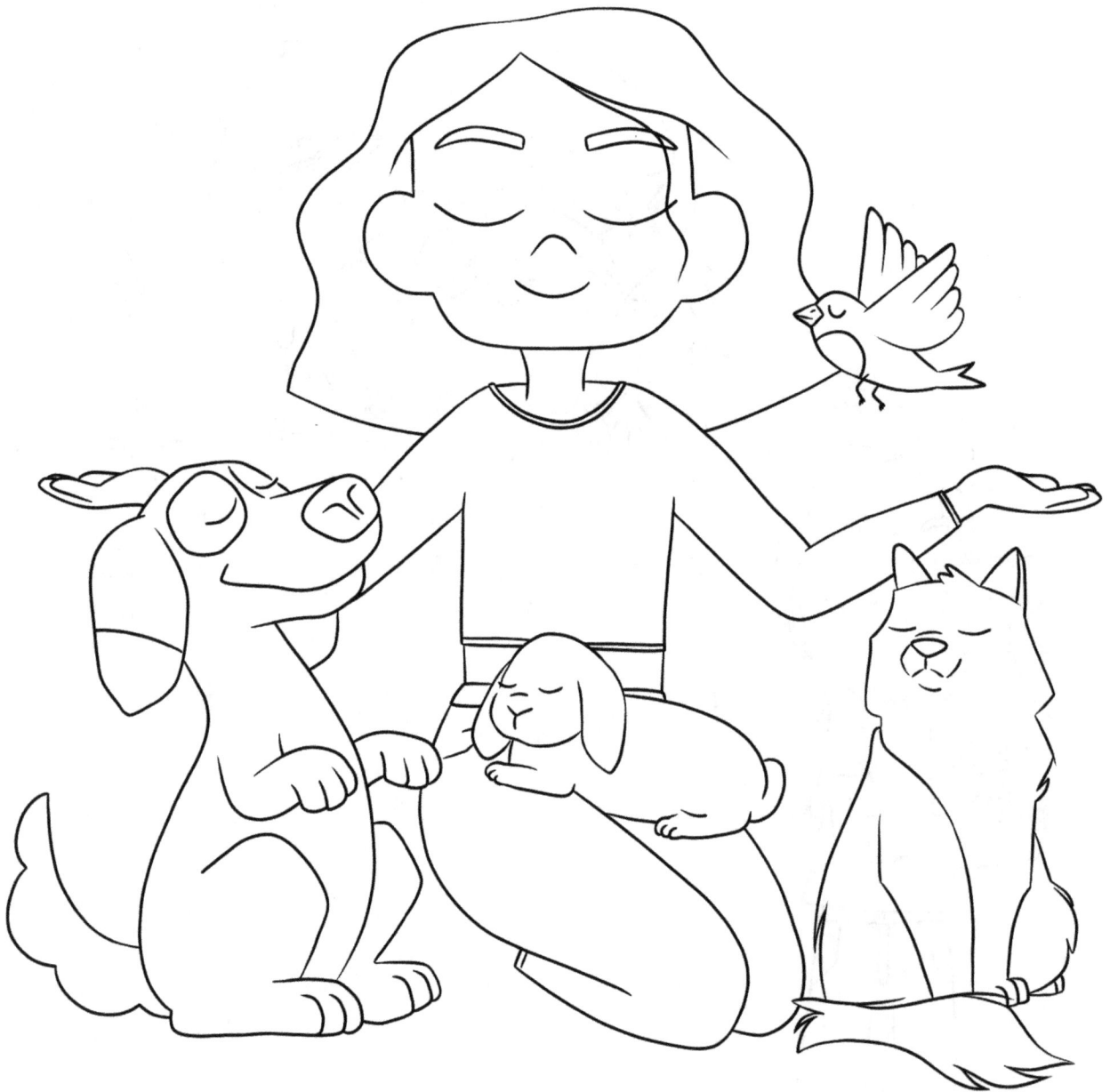

Fluffy Puppy LOVES his Reiki! He can share Reiki too!

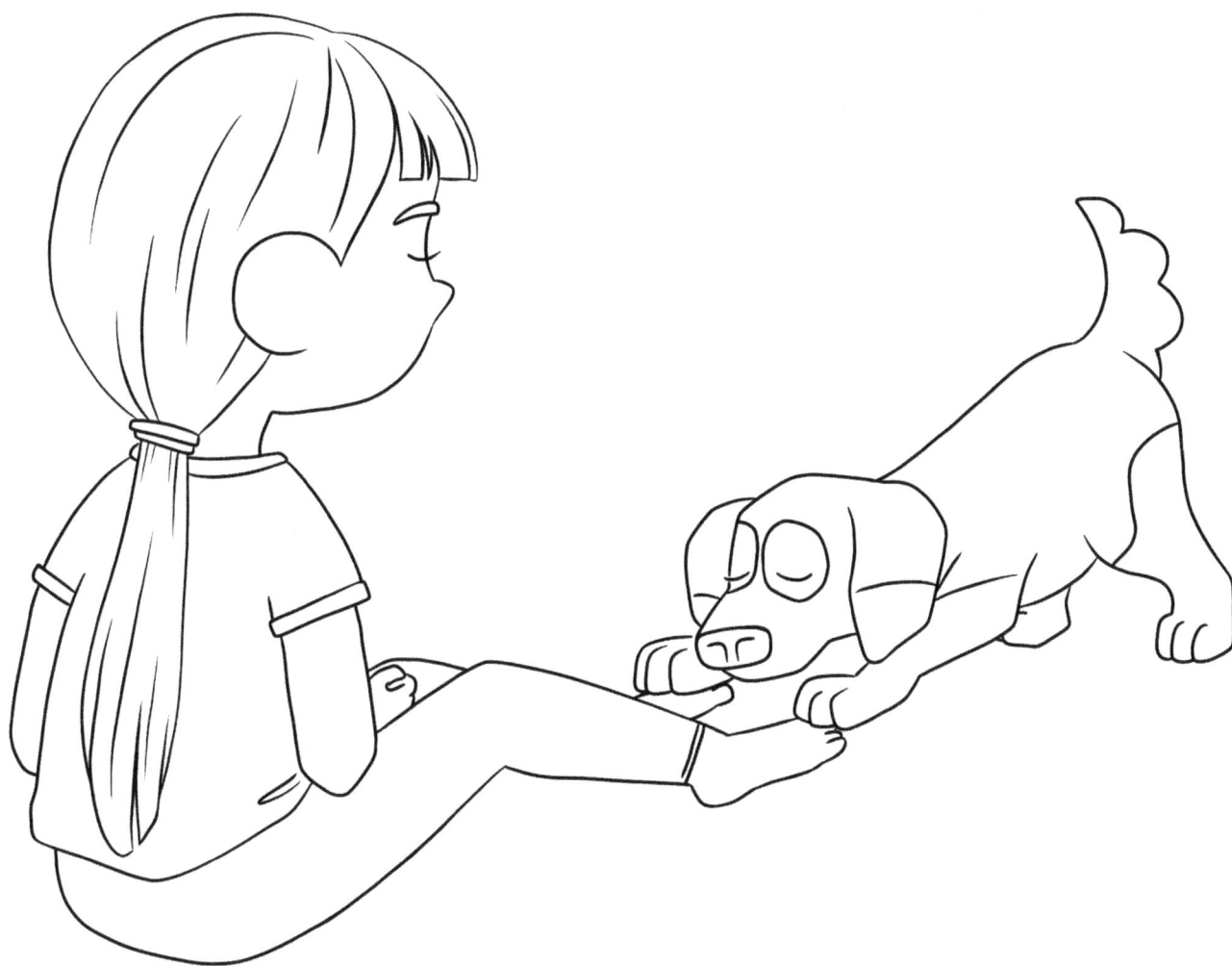

You can even Reiki your food

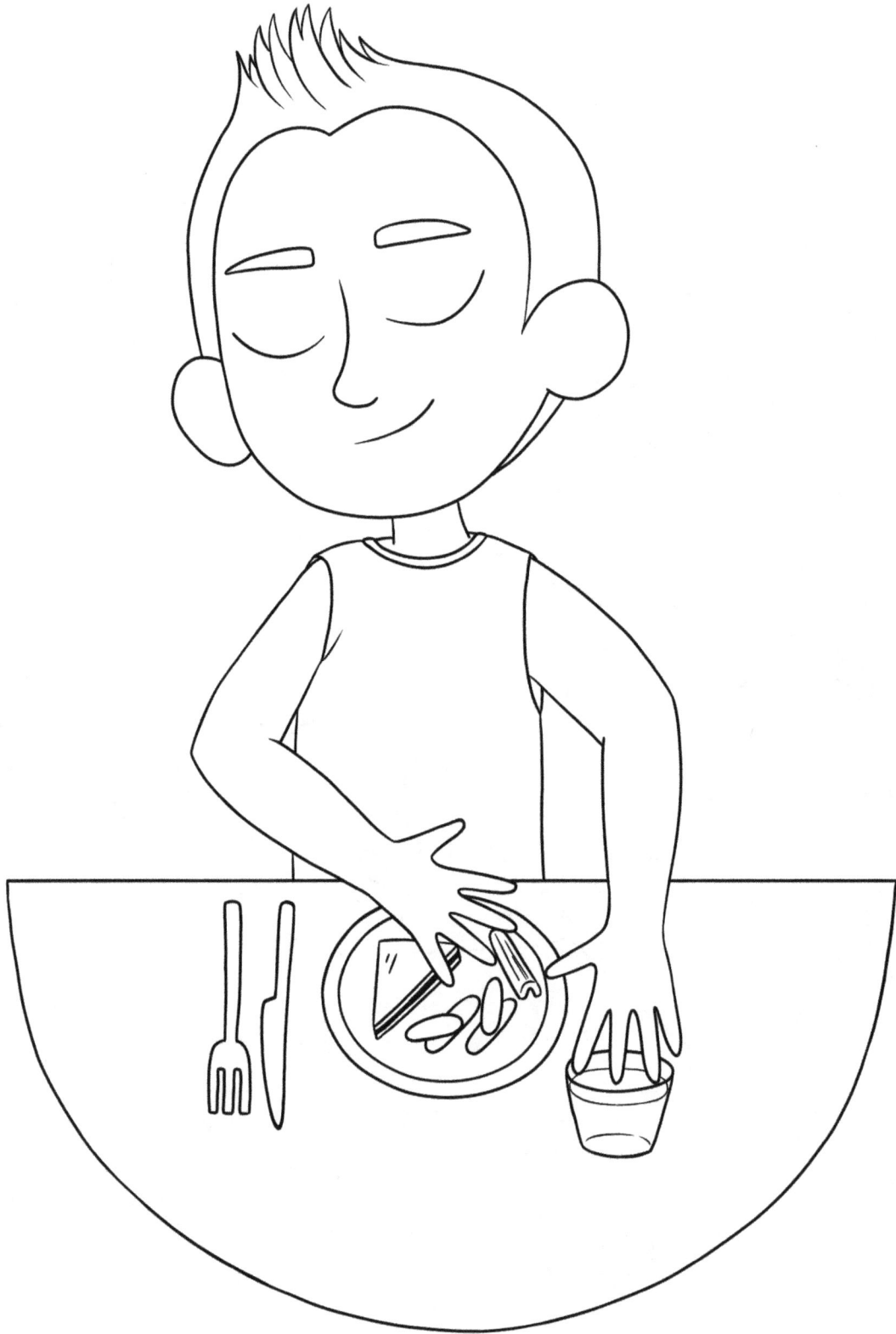

LIVING REIKI EVERYday!

Let's learn the Reiki Rickie Healing Song!

Just for today I don't worry

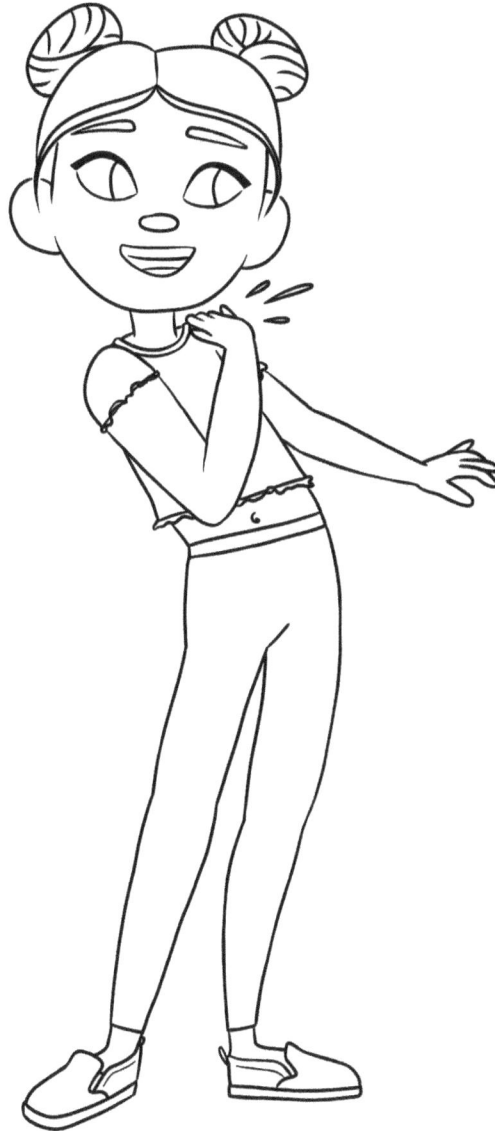

Push those worries away!

Check out our ReikiKids video at ReikibyRickie.com
and sing along with us!

Just for today I am peaceful

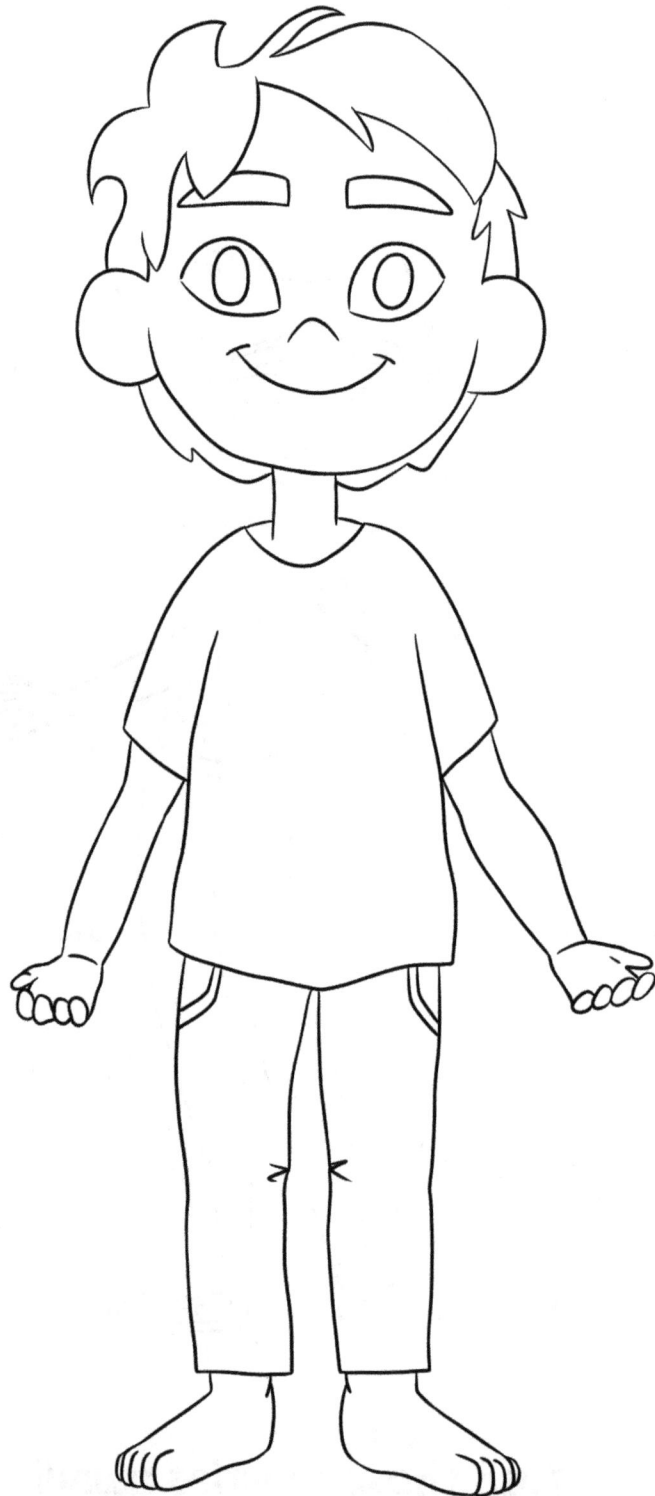

Everyone take a deep breath and say "Ahhhh....."

Just for today I am kind to everyone

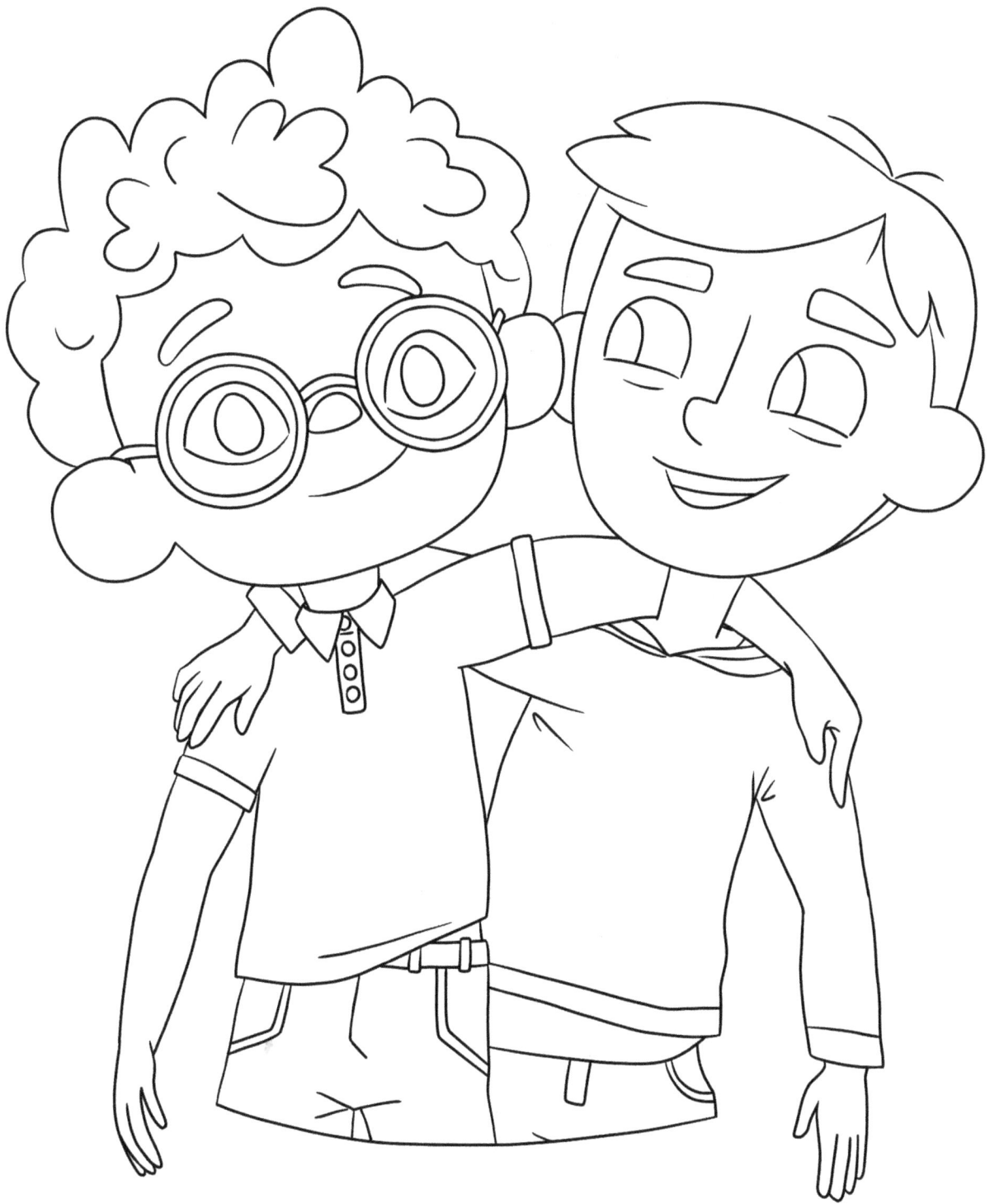

Just for today I work hard

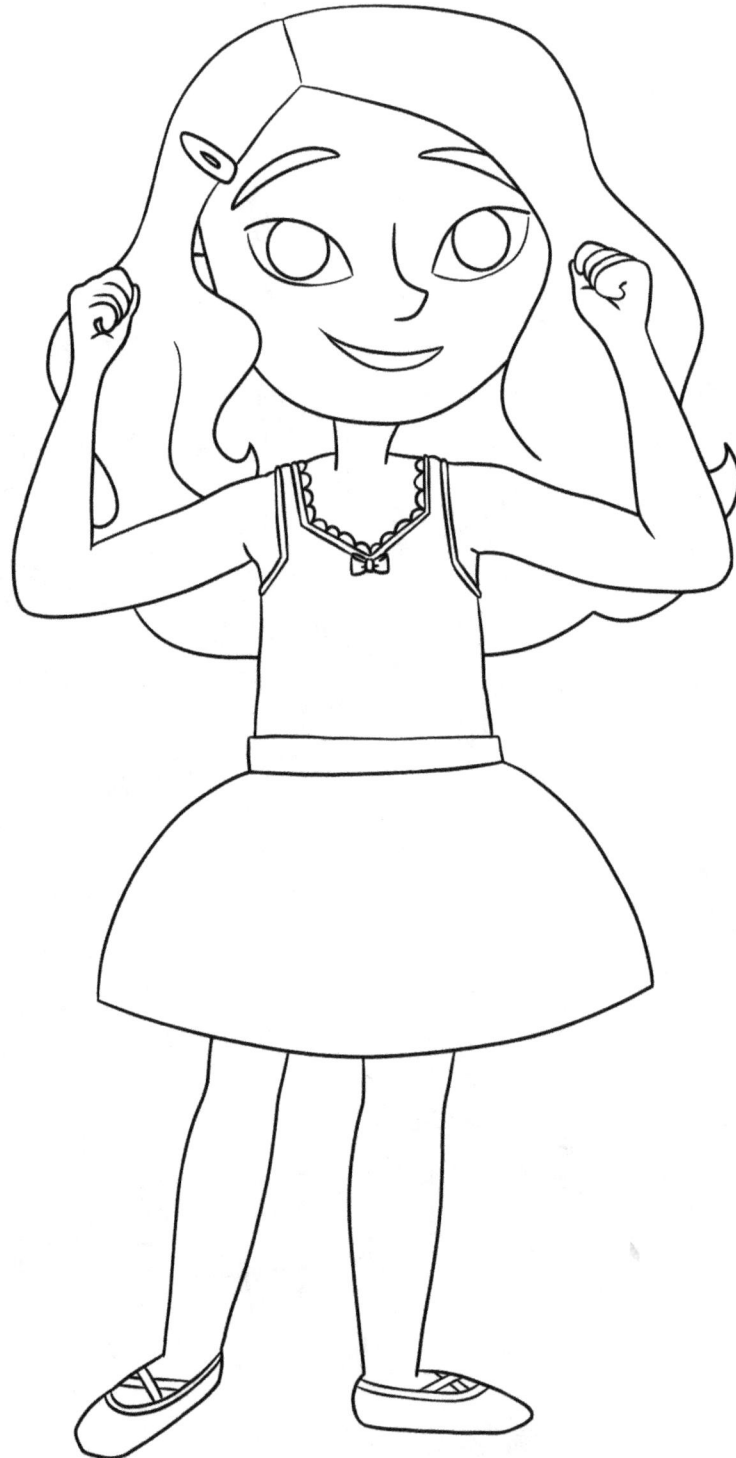

You are strong inside! Grunt and show off your muscles!

Just for today I am grateful...

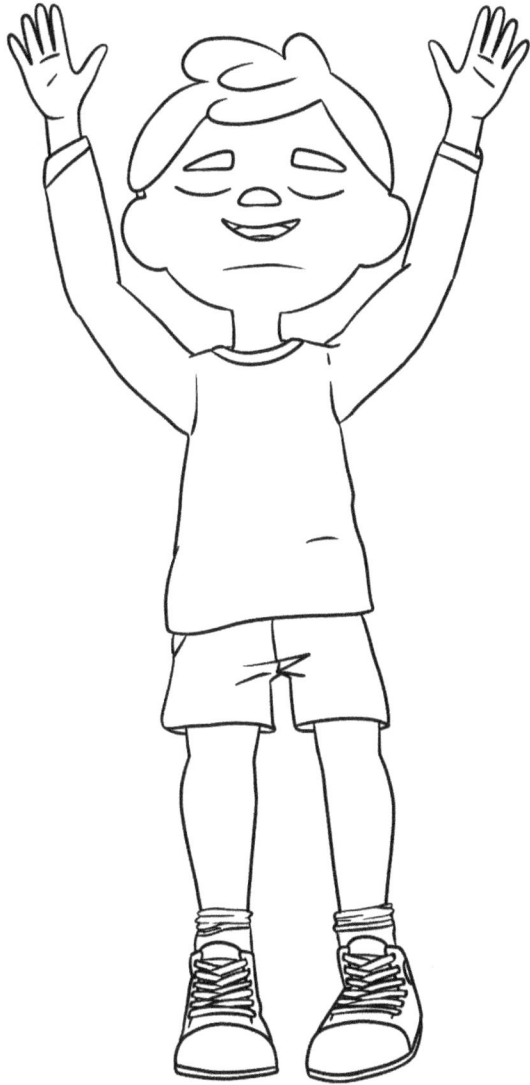

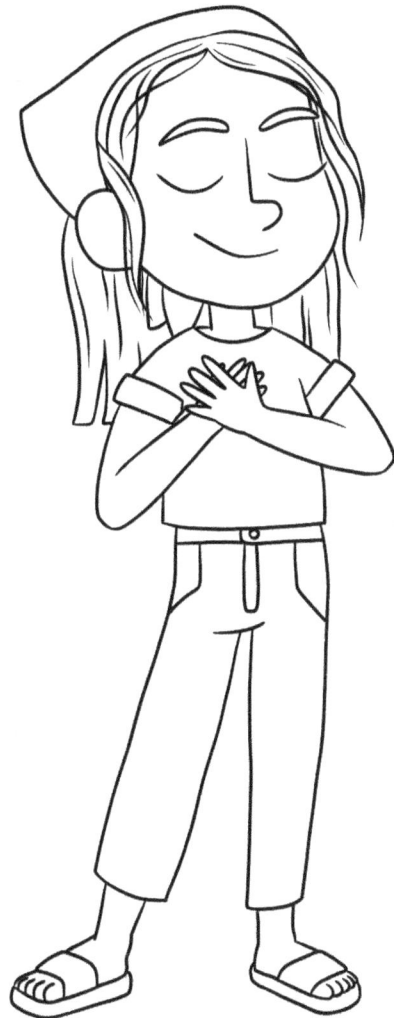

...and loving!

Just for today I am ME!

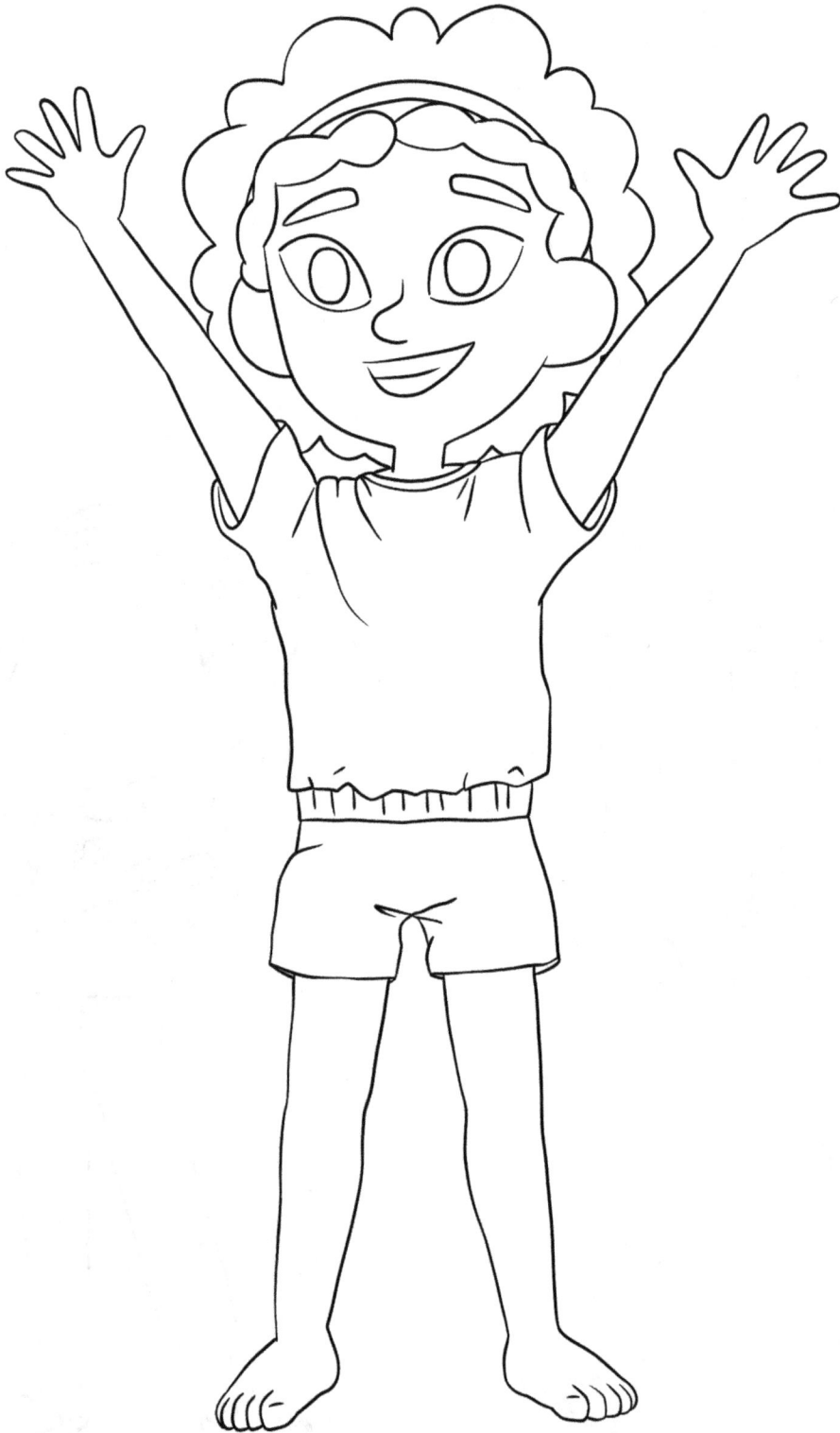

Be your True Self. Let your big, beautiful, bright light SHINE!

What does YOUR energy look and feel like?

DRAW AND COLOR IT HERE

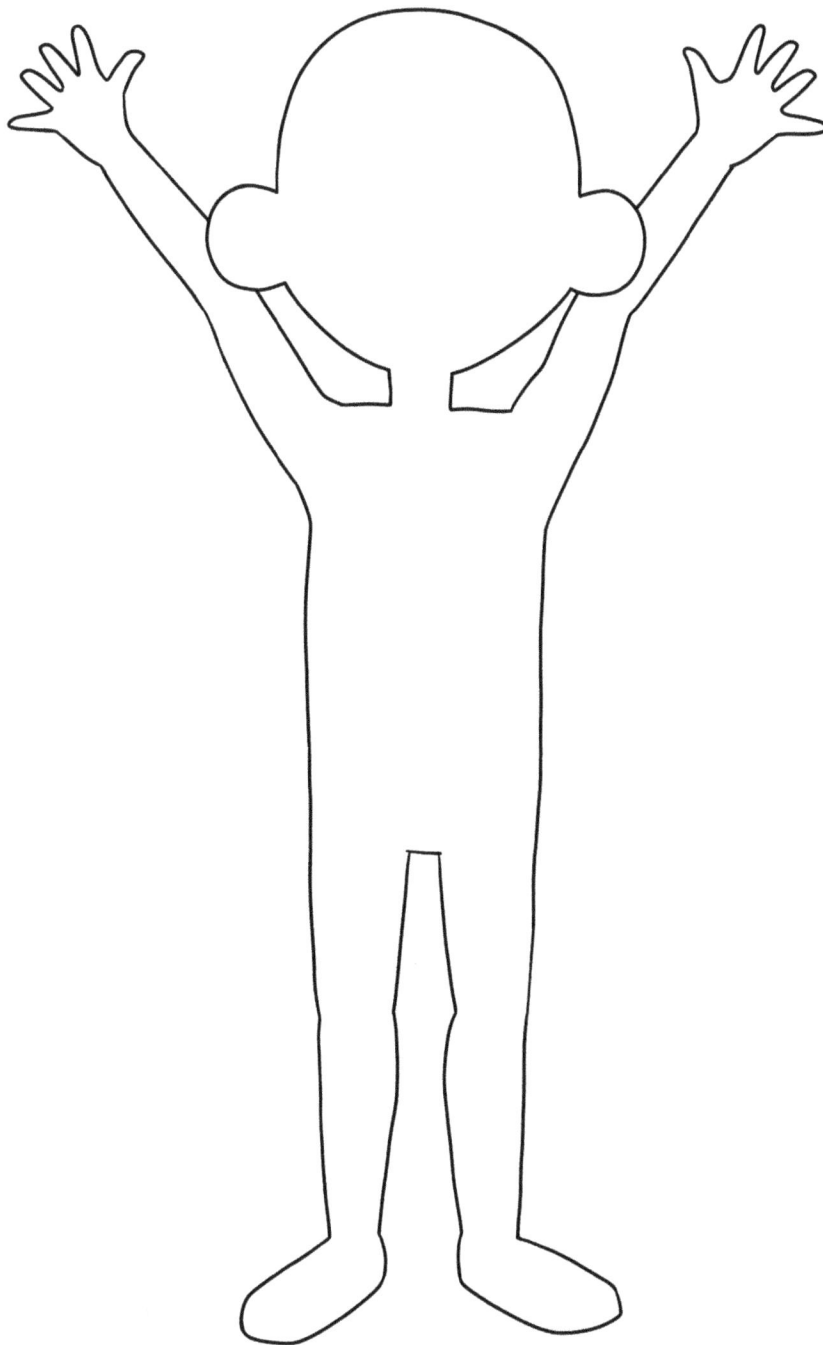